Table of Contents

Introduction
- Welcome and author's introduction
- The significance of addressing menopause
- What to expect from the book

Chapter 1: Understanding Menopause
- Definition of menopause and its stages
- Common symptoms and their causes
- Debunking myths about menopause

Chapter 2: Preparing for the Change
- Recognizing signs of perimenopause
- Emotional and psychological aspects of transitioning
- Lifestyle adjustments to ease the transition

Chapter 3: Managing Hot Flashes
- What are hot flashes and why do they occur?
- Coping strategies for hot flashes (e.g., cooling techniques)
- Herbal remedies and medical treatments

Chapter 4: Hormonal Changes and Their Effects
- The role of hormones during menopause
- Dealing with mood swings, irritability, and other emotional changes
- Hormone replacement therapy (HRT) and its alternatives

Chapter 5: Nutritional Support
- Importance of a balanced diet during menopause
- Foods to alleviate symptoms and promote bone health
- Recipes and meal plans for menopausal women

Chapter 6: Exercise and Physical Health
- The impact of exercise on menopausal symptoms
- Suitable workouts and fitness routines
- Yoga and relaxation techniques

Chapter 7: Mental and Emotional Well-being
- Coping with anxiety, depression, and stress

- Mindfulness and meditation for emotional balance
- Seeking professional help when needed

Chapter 8: Navigating Relationships
- Communicating with loved ones about menopause
- Maintaining intimacy and sexual health
- Building a support network

Chapter 9: Living Your Best Life Beyond Menopause
- Life after menopause - a new beginning
- Rediscovering passions and interests
- Staying healthy and happy in the long term

Conclusion
- Summing up the key takeaways
- Encouraging readers to embrace menopause as a positive life stage
- Providing additional resources and support

Introduction

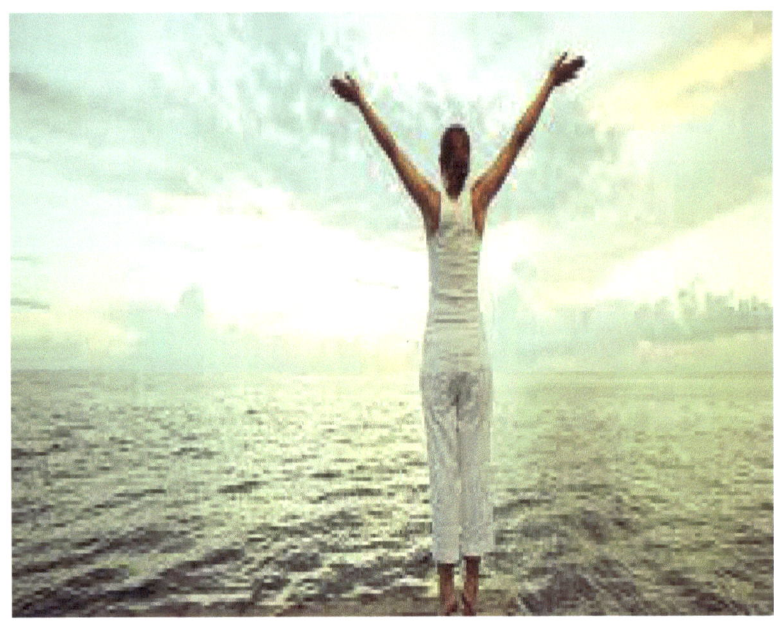

Welcome to "Hot Flashes, Cool Solutions: A Menopause Survival Guide." I'm thrilled to be your guide through this transformative journey. I'm Daniel Watkins, and I understand that menopause can be a challenging and, at times, bewildering phase in a woman's life. It's my passion and privilege to help you navigate these uncharted waters with grace and confidence.

Menopause is not just a biological event; it's a profound life transition that affects us physically, emotionally, and mentally. It's a topic often whispered about, misunderstood, and sometimes even stigmatized. But it's a conversation that must be had, an experience that deserves to be understood, and a phase in your life that can be enriched with knowledge, support, and practical solutions.

In this book, we'll dive deep into the significance of addressing menopause head-on. We'll explore the common symptoms and challenges faced by women during this stage of life, from hot flashes to hormonal fluctuations and everything in between. It's my mission to debunk myths, provide clarity, and empower you with knowledge so that you can embrace this change with a sense of empowerment.

What can you expect from this book? You can anticipate a comprehensive and compassionate guide designed to help you thrive during menopause. We'll cover a wide range of topics, from understanding the biological processes at play to practical tips on managing symptoms, improving your mental and emotional well-being, nurturing your relationships, and ultimately living your best life beyond menopause.

I'm here to be your companion, your source of wisdom, and your confidante throughout this remarkable journey. So, let's embark on this adventure together, and discover the "cool solutions" that can make your menopause experience a more comfortable and fulfilling one.

Chapter 1: Understanding Menopause

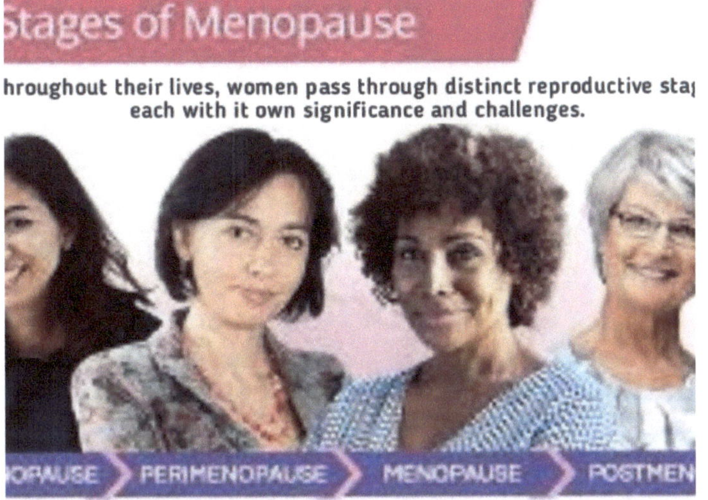

Definition of Menopause and Its Stages

Menopause, often referred to as the "*change of life*," is a natural biological process that marks the end of a woman's reproductive years. It is important to grasp the key aspects of menopause, including its stages. Menopause typically occurs in three primary stages:

1. **Perimenopause**: This is the transitional stage leading up to menopause. It can start in your late 30s or early 40s and may last for several years. During perimenopause, your body begins to produce fewer reproductive hormones, leading to

irregular menstrual cycles and the onset of various symptoms.

2. **Menopause**: Menopause is officially reached when you've gone 12 consecutive months without a menstrual period. The average age for menopause is around 51, but it can happen earlier or later for some women.

3. **Postmenopause**: Postmenopause is the phase of life after menopause. In this stage, the symptoms that were common during perimenopause tend to diminish, although other health considerations become relevant, such as bone health and heart health.

Common Symptoms and Their Causes

Menopause is a unique experience for each woman, but there are several common symptoms you may encounter. These symptoms are primarily caused by the hormonal changes that take place as your body adjusts to lower levels of estrogen and progesterone. Some of the most prevalent symptoms include:

- **Hot Flashes**: Sudden and intense sensations of heat, often accompanied by sweating and a rapid heartbeat. The exact cause is not fully understood, but hormonal fluctuations are a contributing factor.

- **Night Sweats**: Similar to hot flashes but occurring during the night, these can disrupt your sleep patterns.

- **Irregular Periods**: As you approach menopause, your menstrual cycles may become irregular, with varying flow and duration.

- **Vaginal Dryness**: A decrease in estrogen levels can lead to vaginal dryness and discomfort during intercourse.

- **Mood Swings**: Hormonal changes can affect your mood, leading to irritability, anxiety, and even depression in some cases.

- **Sleep Disturbances**: Many women experience difficulty sleeping during menopause, often attributed to night sweats and mood swings.

Debunking Myths About Menopause

Menopause is shrouded in myths and misconceptions that can add unnecessary anxiety to this already challenging phase of life. Let's take a moment to debunk some of these common myths:

Myth 1: Menopause Is a Disease: Menopause is not an illness or a disease. It's a natural, biological process that every woman experiences as she gets older.

Myth 2: Menopause Means the End of Intimacy: While menopause can bring about changes in sexual function, it doesn't mean the end of intimacy. There are solutions and strategies to maintain a healthy and fulfilling sex life.

Myth 3: Menopause Starts at a Fixed Age: Menopause is highly individual, and the age at which it begins can vary greatly. It's not solely determined by reaching a specific number.

Myth 4: All Menopause Symptoms Are Severe: Not all women experience severe symptoms. Some may go through menopause with minimal discomfort, while others may have more pronounced symptoms.

Understanding the stages, common symptoms, and dispelling these myths is a crucial step toward navigating the challenges of menopause with confidence and knowledge. In the following chapters, we'll explore strategies and solutions to make this journey more manageable and even empowering.

Chapter 2: Preparing for the Change

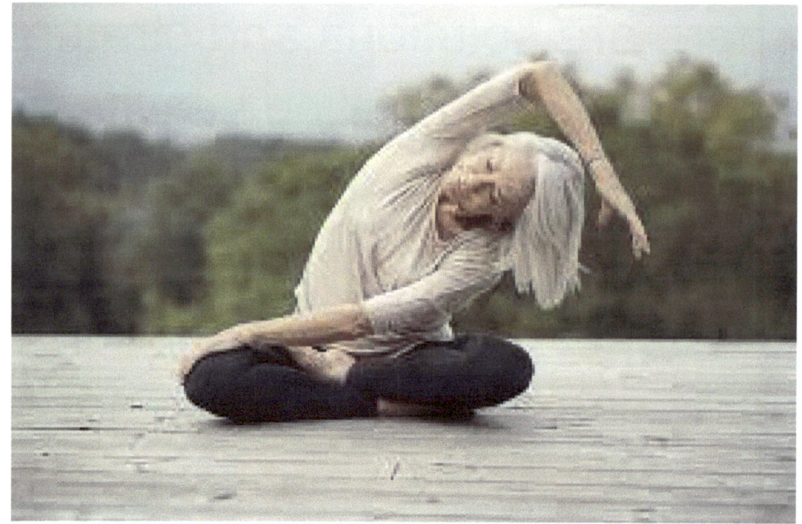

Recognizing Signs of Perimenopause

Perimenopause is a significant part of your journey toward menopause, and recognizing its signs is crucial for understanding the changes your body is undergoing. Here are some common signs to look out for:

1. **Irregular Periods**: Your menstrual cycle may become unpredictable, with variations in flow and duration.

2. **Hot Flashes**: While hot flashes can be a symptom of full menopause, they often begin during perimenopause.

3. **Mood Swings**: Hormonal fluctuations can lead to mood swings, irritability, and increased emotional sensitivity.

4. **Sleep Disturbances**: You might start experiencing difficulties with sleep, such as night sweats or insomnia.

5. **Changes in Libido**: Some women notice changes in sexual desire or discomfort during intercourse.

6. **Vaginal Changes**: Vaginal dryness, itching, and discomfort can occur due to reduced estrogen levels.

Emotional and Psychological Aspects of Transitioning

The transition into menopause isn't only physical; it's a deeply emotional and psychological journey as well. It's essential to acknowledge and address the emotional aspects of this transition:

- **Acceptance**: Understand that this is a natural phase of life. Embrace it as a new chapter rather than a loss of youth or fertility.

- **Self-Reflection**: Take time to reflect on your feelings and thoughts about menopause. This can help you process the changes more effectively.

- **Communication**: Openly discuss your experiences and concerns with friends, family, or a healthcare professional. Sharing your feelings can provide valuable emotional support.

- **Mental Health**: Prioritize your mental well-being. Practices like mindfulness, meditation, or counseling can help you manage mood swings and anxiety.

- **Self-Care**: Incorporate self-care routines into your daily life. Simple acts of self-compassion, like taking a relaxing bath, reading, or pursuing hobbies, can do wonders for your emotional health.

Lifestyle Adjustments to Ease the Transition

Your lifestyle plays a significant role in how you experience perimenopause and menopause. Making some thoughtful adjustments can greatly ease the transition:

1. **Nutrition**: A balanced diet rich in fruits, vegetables, and whole grains can help manage symptoms. Foods containing phytoestrogens, like soy and flaxseeds, can be beneficial.

2. **Exercise**: Regular physical activity, such as walking, swimming, or yoga, can help maintain a healthy weight and alleviate symptoms like hot flashes.

3. **Stress Management**: Stress can exacerbate menopausal symptoms. Explore stress-reduction

techniques like deep breathing, progressive muscle relaxation, or meditation.

4. **Sleep Hygiene**: Prioritize good sleep hygiene, which includes maintaining a consistent sleep schedule, creating a comfortable sleep environment, and limiting caffeine and electronics before bedtime.

5. **Hormone Replacement Therapy (HRT)**: If you're considering HRT, discuss the benefits and risks with your healthcare provider. It can be a suitable option for some women.

Preparation for perimenopause is about embracing the changes, both physical and emotional, and making proactive choices to ease the transition. In the chapters that follow, we will delve deeper into practical strategies for managing specific symptoms and improving your overall well-being during this transformative time.

Chapter 3: Managing Hot Flashes

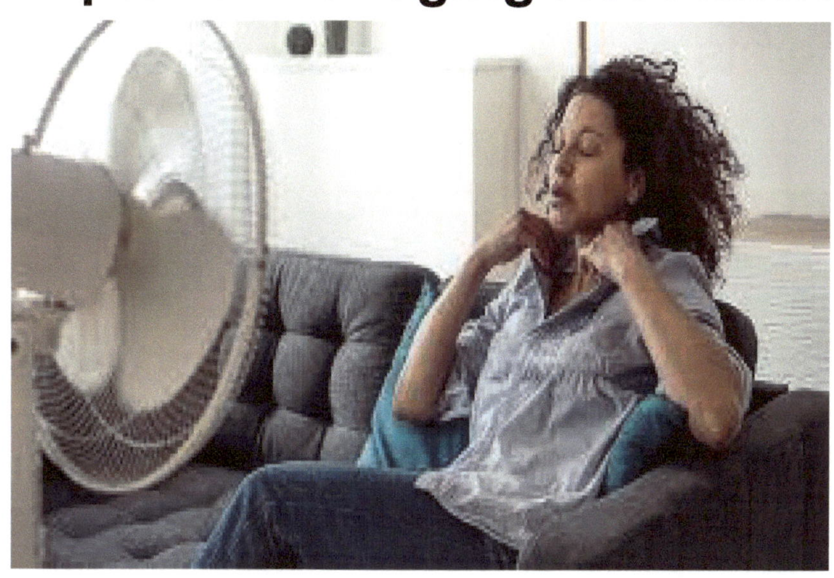

What Are Hot Flashes and Why Do They Occur?

Hot flashes are perhaps the most notorious and disruptive symptom of menopause. They are characterized by sudden, intense sensations of heat, often accompanied by sweating and a rapid heartbeat. Understanding why hot flashes occur is essential:

 Hormonal Imbalance: The primary cause of hot flashes is the hormonal changes that come with menopause. Fluctuations in estrogen levels can confuse the body's internal thermostat, leading to sudden bursts of heat.

 Vasomotor Instability: These hormonal changes can disrupt the function of blood vessels, causing them to dilate (widen) and contract (narrow) abruptly. This rapid fluctuation in blood flow can lead to the sensation of heat.

 Triggers: Certain factors, such as stress, spicy foods, caffeine, alcohol, and smoking, can trigger or exacerbate hot flashes.

Coping Strategies for Hot Flashes (e.g., Cooling Techniques)

Dealing with hot flashes can be challenging, but there are numerous coping strategies that can help you regain control and find relief:

1. **Dress in Layers**: Wear lightweight, breathable clothing in layers so you can easily remove items when a hot flash strikes.

2. **Stay Cool**: Keep your environment comfortably cool by using fans, opening windows, or using air conditioning. Sleeping with breathable sheets and blankets can also help.

3. **Deep Breathing**: Practice deep, slow breathing when a hot flash begins. Deep breaths can help calm your body's response to the sensation.

4. **Cooling Techniques**: Apply a cool, damp cloth to your forehead or the back of your neck during a hot flash. Some women find handheld fans or cooling sprays helpful.

5. **Stay Hydrated**: Drink plenty of water throughout the day to help regulate body temperature. Avoid caffeine and alcohol, as they can trigger hot flashes.

6. **Stress Reduction**: Techniques like yoga, meditation, and mindfulness can reduce stress

and potentially decrease the frequency and intensity of hot flashes.

7. **Biofeedback**: Some women find relief through biofeedback therapy, which helps control physiological responses to stress.

8. **Acupuncture**: Acupuncture has been shown to alleviate hot flashes for some women.

Herbal Remedies and Medical Treatments

Herbal remedies and medical treatments offer a range of options for managing hot flashes:

Herbal Remedies: Certain herbal supplements, like black cohosh and evening primrose oil, have been used to alleviate menopausal symptoms. However, results can vary, and it's essential to consult with a healthcare provider before using any herbal remedy.

Hormone Replacement Therapy (HRT): HRT is a medical treatment involving the use of estrogen and, sometimes, progestin to alleviate menopausal symptoms, including hot flashes. It can be highly effective, but it's essential to discuss the benefits and risks with your healthcare provider.

Non-Hormonal Medications: Some non-hormonal medications, such as selective serotonin reuptake inhibitors (SSRIs) and serotonin-norepinephrine reuptake inhibitors (SNRIs), may be prescribed to manage hot flashes.

Medical Devices: Certain medical devices, such as the Brisdelle capsule, can be used to manage hot flashes.

This chapter provides you with the knowledge and practical strategies to manage hot flashes effectively. Remember that the best approach may vary from person to person, so it's important to consult with a healthcare provider to determine the most suitable solutions for your individual needs.

Chapter 4: Hormonal Changes and Their Effects

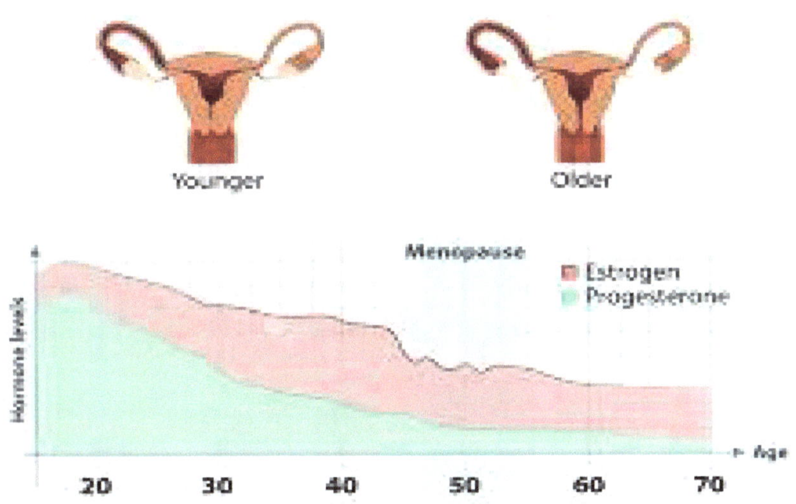

The Role of Hormones During Menopause

Hormones are the conductors of the intricate symphony that is your body's physiology, and during menopause, this symphony experiences a significant shift. Understanding the role of hormones during this phase is essential:

Estrogen: Estrogen, a hormone primarily produced by the ovaries, plays a pivotal role in a woman's reproductive and overall health. During menopause, estrogen levels decline, leading to various physical and emotional changes.

 Progesterone: Progesterone, another ovarian hormone, helps regulate the menstrual cycle. Its levels also decrease during menopause.

 Follicle-Stimulating Hormone (FSH): FSH levels rise as the body attempts to stimulate the ovaries to produce more estrogen. Elevated FSH levels are a hallmark of menopause.

Dealing with Mood Swings, Irritability, and Other Emotional Changes

Hormonal changes during menopause can have a profound impact on your emotional well-being. You may experience mood swings, irritability, and emotional turbulence. Here's how to manage these changes:

1. **Recognize the Source**: Understanding that these emotions are often hormonally driven can

help you detach from them and better manage your reactions.

2. **Seek Emotional Support**: Share your feelings with loved ones or a mental health professional. They can provide understanding and guidance during challenging emotional moments.

3. **Practice Stress Reduction**: Stress can amplify emotional turmoil. Engage in stress-reduction techniques like mindfulness, yoga, or meditation.

4. **Maintain a Healthy Lifestyle**: Regular exercise, a balanced diet, and adequate sleep can have a positive impact on your mood.

5. **Hormone Replacement Therapy (HRT) and Its Alternatives**

Hormone Replacement Therapy (HRT) is a common approach to alleviate menopausal symptoms, including mood swings. Here's what you need to know about HRT and its alternatives:

Hormone Replacement Therapy (HRT): HRT involves the use of estrogen and, in some cases, progestin to replace the hormones your body is no longer producing at premenopausal levels. It can effectively manage mood swings, hot flashes, and other symptoms.

Benefits of HRT: HRT can relieve severe menopausal symptoms, reduce the risk of osteoporosis, and potentially improve mood.

Risks of HRT: HRT is not suitable for everyone and carries some risks, such as an increased risk of blood clots, stroke, and breast cancer. It's essential to discuss the benefits and risks with your healthcare provider.

Alternatives to HRT: For those who cannot or do not want to use HRT, there are alternative treatments and strategies, such as lifestyle changes, herbal remedies, and non-hormonal medications. These options may help manage mood swings and other symptoms.

Managing hormonal changes and their emotional effects during menopause can be challenging, but with the right knowledge and support, it's entirely possible. In the chapters ahead, we'll delve deeper into strategies for navigating these changes with grace and confidence.

Chapter 5: Nutritional Support

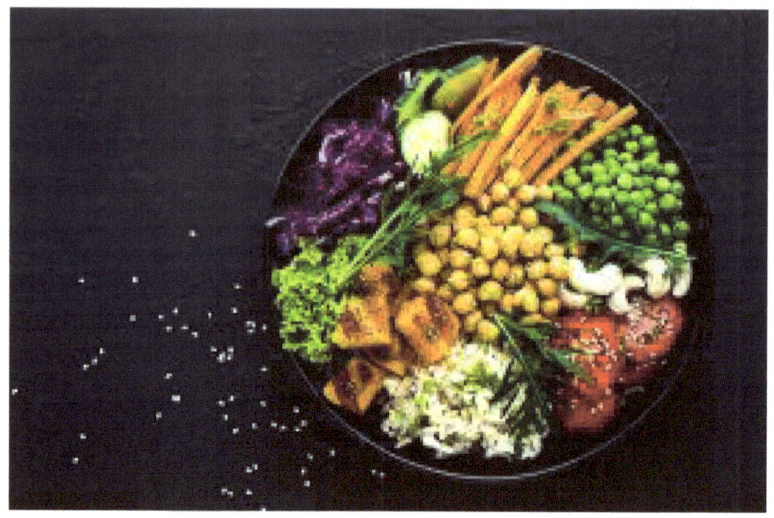

Importance of a Balanced Diet During Menopause

Menopause is a time of significant change in a woman's life, and proper nutrition is essential to support your physical and emotional well-being during this transition. Here, we'll explore the importance of maintaining a balanced diet during menopause:

Hormonal Balance: A balanced diet helps stabilize hormone levels, reducing the severity of symptoms like hot flashes and mood swings.

Bone Health: Menopause is associated with a decline in bone density. A diet rich in essential nutrients can help maintain bone health and reduce the risk of osteoporosis.

Heart Health: As estrogen levels decrease, the risk of heart disease increases. A heart-healthy diet can mitigate this risk.

Foods to Alleviate Symptoms and Promote Bone Health

Specific foods can play a significant role in alleviating menopausal symptoms and supporting bone health:

Calcium-Rich Foods: Dairy products, leafy green vegetables, and fortified non-dairy alternatives are excellent sources of calcium, which is vital for maintaining bone strength.

Vitamin D: Your body needs vitamin D to absorb calcium. You can get it from fatty fish, eggs, and fortified foods, or through safe sun exposure.

Phytoestrogenic Foods: Foods containing natural plant compounds, such as soy products and flaxseeds, mimic the effects of estrogen and can help reduce menopausal symptoms.

Healthy Fats: Omega-3 fatty acids, found in fatty fish like salmon and walnuts, support heart health and reduce inflammation.

Fiber-Rich Foods: Whole grains, fruits, and vegetables high in fiber can aid in managing weight, stabilizing blood sugar, and promoting digestive health.

Recipes and Meal Plans for Menopausal Women

Eating well during menopause doesn't have to be a challenge. Consider these sample recipes and meal plans designed to support women during this phase:

1. **Breakfast**: A Greek yogurt parfait with berries, nuts, and honey, accompanied by whole-grain toast and a glass of fresh orange juice.

2. **Lunch**: A quinoa and roasted vegetable salad with a side of hummus and whole-grain crackers.

3. **Snack**: Sliced apple with almond butter or a small serving of mixed nuts.

4. **Dinner**: Baked salmon with a side of quinoa and steamed broccoli, followed by a mixed-berry dessert.

5. **Vegetarian Option**: A spinach and chickpea curry served with brown rice and a fresh cucumber and tomato salad.

6. **Vegan Option**: A hearty lentil stew with plenty of vegetables and a side of whole-grain bread.

These meal ideas provide a balanced mix of nutrients, including calcium, vitamin D, phytoestrogens, and omega-3 fatty acids, all of which can help manage menopausal symptoms and support your overall health.

A well-planned diet can make a significant difference in how you experience menopause. With the right nutritional support, you can navigate this transition with vitality and well-being. In the chapters ahead, we'll explore more strategies for thriving during this transformative period.

Chapter 6: Exercise and Physical Health

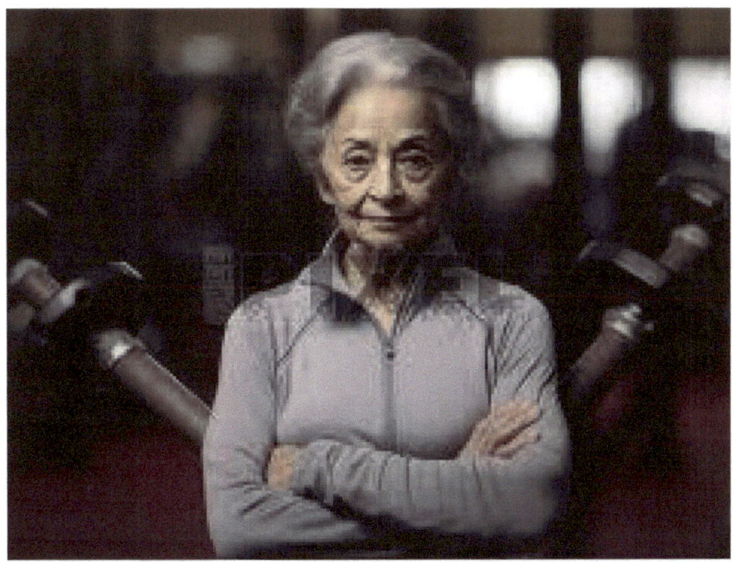

The Impact of Exercise on Menopausal Symptoms

Regular physical activity is a powerful tool for managing menopausal symptoms and promoting overall well-being. Let's explore the significant impact exercise has on your journey through menopause:

- **Hot Flashes**: Exercise can help reduce the frequency and intensity of hot flashes by regulating your body's thermostat.

- **Mood and Emotional Health**: Physical activity releases endorphins, which can help combat mood swings, irritability, and depression commonly associated with menopause.

- **Weight Management**: Menopause often brings changes in metabolism and weight gain. Exercise can assist in maintaining a healthy weight.

- **Bone Health**: Weight-bearing exercises like walking and resistance training help strengthen bones, reducing the risk of osteoporosis.

Suitable Workouts and Fitness Routines

The right workouts and routines can make a substantial difference in managing menopausal symptoms. Consider these options:

1. **Aerobic Exercise**: Activities like brisk walking, jogging, swimming, and dancing improve cardiovascular health and help manage weight.

2. **Strength Training**: Resistance exercises with weights, resistance bands, or body weight can maintain and increase muscle mass, essential for overall strength and bone health.

3. **Flexibility Exercises:** Yoga and Pilates enhance flexibility and balance, reducing the risk of injury and improving overall well-being.

4. **Mind-Body Exercises**: Mindfulness-based exercises, such as tai chi, promote relaxation and emotional well-being.

5. **Interval Training**: This involves alternating between high-intensity and low-intensity exercise and can be highly effective for managing weight and reducing hot flashes.

Yoga and Relaxation Techniques

Yoga, in particular, can be a valuable addition to your menopause journey. It not only enhances physical health but also provides relaxation techniques for emotional and psychological well-being:

1. **Deep Breathing**: Yoga encourages deep, mindful breathing, which can help manage stress, reduce anxiety, and regulate mood swings.

2. **Stress Reduction**: The practice of yoga involves relaxation and mindfulness techniques that can effectively reduce stress and enhance emotional stability.

3. **Balance and Flexibility**: Yoga poses can improve balance and flexibility, reducing the risk of falls and enhancing overall physical health.

4. **Emotional Support**: Joining a yoga class or community can provide emotional support and a

sense of belonging during this transformative time.

Incorporating exercise and relaxation techniques into your daily routine can significantly enhance your physical and emotional well-being during menopause. In the upcoming chapters, we'll delve into even more strategies and solutions to make your menopause journey as comfortable and fulfilling as possible.

Chapter 7: Mental and Emotional Well-being

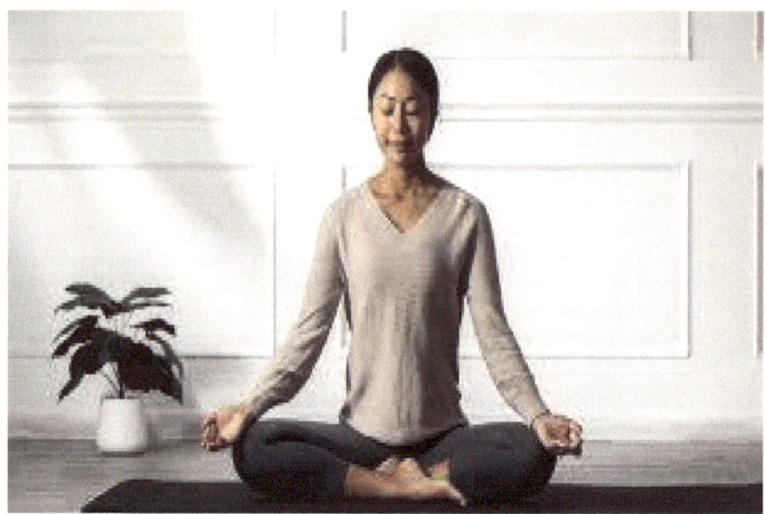

Coping with Anxiety, Depression, and Stress

Menopause is not just a physical journey; it's also a mental and emotional one. It's common for women to experience heightened anxiety, depression, and stress during this time. Here's how to cope with these challenges:

1. **Recognize the Signs**: Acknowledge the symptoms of anxiety and depression, such as persistent sadness, mood swings, and intense worry.

2. **Mindful Awareness**: Start by becoming more aware of your thoughts and emotions. This

self-awareness can help you identify patterns and triggers for anxiety and stress.

3. **Support System**: Lean on your support network, including friends and family, and talk about your feelings. Sharing your concerns can provide emotional relief.

4. **Stress Management**: Engage in stress-reduction techniques like deep breathing exercises, progressive muscle relaxation, or journaling to unload your thoughts and emotions.

Mindfulness and Meditation for Emotional Balance

Practicing mindfulness and meditation can be transformative in managing your emotional well-being during menopause:

1. **Mindfulness Meditation**: This practice involves paying attention to the present moment without judgment. It can help reduce anxiety,

promote emotional balance, and improve overall well-being.

2. **Guided Meditation**: Follow guided meditation sessions or apps designed for stress reduction, relaxation, and emotional stability.

3. **Yoga and Tai Chi**: These activities combine mindfulness with physical movements, offering a holistic approach to emotional balance.

4. **Breathing Exercises**: Incorporate simple deep-breathing exercises into your daily routine. They can calm your mind and reduce anxiety.

Seeking Professional Help When Needed

Sometimes, managing menopausal emotions may require professional guidance. Don't hesitate to seek help when needed:

1. **Therapy**: A mental health professional can provide therapy, such as cognitive-behavioral

therapy (CBT), to address anxiety and depression.

2. **Medication**: In some cases, medication may be necessary to manage severe anxiety or depression. Discuss this option with a healthcare provider.

3. **Support Groups**: Joining a menopause support group can provide a safe space to share experiences and gain insights from others going through similar challenges.

4. **Counseling**: A counselor or therapist can help you navigate the emotional and psychological aspects of menopause.

Remember that seeking professional help is a sign of strength and self-care. It's essential to prioritize your mental and emotional well-being as much as your physical health during this transformative phase of life.

In the following chapters, we'll continue to explore strategies and solutions that will empower you to thrive during menopause. Your journey should be characterized not only by survival but by growth and fulfillment.

Chapter 8: Navigating Relationships

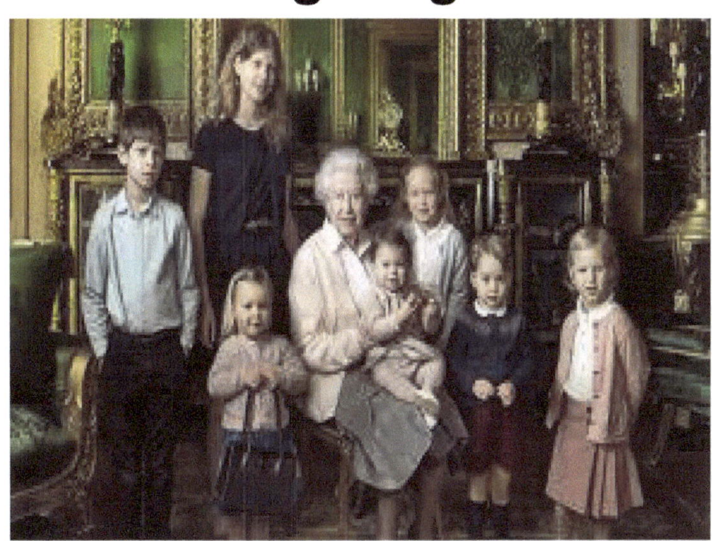

Communicating with Loved Ones About Menopause

The menopausal journey doesn't happen in isolation; it can have a significant impact on your relationships with loved ones. Effective communication is vital:

1. **Honesty**: Open, honest communication about what you're experiencing can help your loved ones understand and support you better.

2. **Educate Them**: Share information about menopause, its symptoms, and its impact. The more they know, the better they can empathize.

3. **Ask for Support**: Let your loved ones know what kind of support you need, whether it's a listening ear, help with household chores, or understanding during mood swings.

Maintaining Intimacy and Sexual Health

Menopause can affect your sexual health and intimacy with your partner. Here's how to navigate this aspect of your relationship:

1. **Communication**: Talk to your partner openly about changes in your libido, discomfort, or other sexual issues. An empathetic conversation can bring you closer.

2. **Explore Together**: Experiment with new ways to maintain intimacy, such as trying different forms of physical touch, massage, or simply spending quality time together.

3. **Professional Help**: If needed, consider seeking advice from a healthcare provider or therapist to address specific sexual health concerns.

Building a Support Network

Menopause is a shared experience among countless women. Building a support network can provide invaluable emotional backing:

1. **Join Support Groups**: Participating in menopause support groups or online communities can connect you with others going through similar experiences.

2. **Friendships**: Maintain and strengthen your friendships with people who understand and support your journey.

3. **Family**: Don't hesitate to lean on family members for support. Sometimes, just knowing

they're there for you can make a significant difference.

4. **Professional Support**: Consider therapy or counseling if the emotional and psychological aspects of menopause become overwhelming. A professional can help you navigate these challenges.

Navigating relationships during menopause is about fostering understanding, maintaining intimacy, and creating a robust support system. As you proceed through this transformative phase, remember that the people who care about you are essential pillars of strength and comfort. In the chapters ahead, we'll delve even deeper into strategies to make this journey as positive and fulfilling as possible.

Chapter 9: Living Your Best Life Beyond Menopause

Life After Menopause - A New Beginning

Menopause is not an end; it's a new beginning. As your body settles into its postmenopausal phase, you'll discover newfound freedom and opportunities. Here's how to embrace this new chapter:

1. **Self-Discovery**: Take time to reacquaint yourself with who you are and what you desire now that menopause has passed. Reflect on your goals and dreams, both old and new.

2. **Reevaluate Your Priorities**: Menopause often prompts a shift in your priorities. Embrace the chance to reprioritize what truly matters to you.

3. **Set New Goals:** Establish fresh aspirations for this stage of life. Whether it's a career change, travel, or pursuing a lifelong hobby, you have the freedom to set new goals.

Rediscovering Passions and Interests

As you transition into postmenopause, it's the perfect time to reconnect with your passions and interests:

1. **Hobbies**: Rediscover hobbies or interests you may have put aside during your busy years. Engaging in hobbies can be a source of joy and fulfillment.

2. **Education**: Consider taking up a new skill or furthering your education. Lifelong learning can invigorate your mind and open new doors.

3. **Travel**: Explore the world. Traveling can be an enriching experience that broadens your horizons and creates lasting memories.

Staying Healthy and Happy in the Long Term

Staying healthy and happy as you age is a priority for many women. Here's how to do it:

1. **Physical Health:** Continue to maintain a balanced diet, engage in regular exercise, and attend routine check-ups with your healthcare provider.

2. **Mental and Emotional Health:** Prioritize emotional well-being through practices like mindfulness, meditation, and therapy. Cultivate a positive mindset to navigate life's challenges.

3. **Social Connections**: Stay socially active. Building and maintaining connections with friends

and family can enhance your happiness and emotional well-being.

4. **Continual Growth:** Keep learning and growing throughout your life. It's never too late to take on new challenges and explore your potential.

5. **Preventative Health:** Maintain regular health screenings, such as mammograms, bone density tests, and heart health check-ups, to detect and prevent potential health issues.

Menopause doesn't signify the end of your life; it marks the beginning of a new and exciting chapter. By embracing change, rediscovering your passions, and nurturing your physical and emotional well-being, you can create a fulfilling and vibrant postmenopausal life. This is your time to shine and celebrate the incredible journey you've undertaken. In this book, we've explored various strategies and solutions to help you thrive during menopause. It's now your opportunity to live your best life beyond menopause.

Chapter 10: Embracing Menopause: A New Beginning

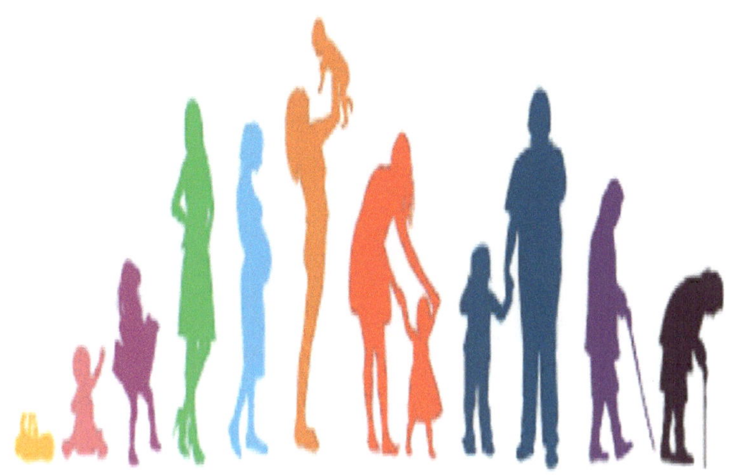

Summing Up the Key Takeaways

As we conclude this guide, let's recap the essential lessons and insights you've gained throughout your journey of "Hot Flashes, Cool Solutions: A Menopause Survival Guide." We've explored various aspects of menopause, from understanding the physical changes to managing emotional well-being, nurturing relationships, and planning for life beyond this transformative phase.

Here are the key takeaways:

1. **Understanding Menopause:** Recognize the stages and symptoms of menopause, debunk myths, and be informed about the changes happening in your body.

2. **Physical Well-being:** Prioritize nutrition, exercise, and rest to manage symptoms and promote your physical health.

3. **Emotional Well-being:** Practice mindfulness, meditation, and seek support when needed to maintain emotional balance.

4. **Relationships**: Communicate openly with loved ones, maintain intimacy, and build a support network that can help you navigate menopause with ease.

5. **Life Beyond Menopause:** Embrace this new chapter, rediscover your passions, and prioritize long-term health and happiness.

Encouraging Readers to Embrace Menopause as a Positive Life Stage

Menopause is not the end; it's a significant beginning. It's a phase that signifies wisdom, strength, and the freedom to shape your life exactly how you want it. Embrace it as a positive life stage, and remember:

- **You Are Not Alone**: Many women are going through this journey with you. Seek support and understanding from your community, friends, and family.

- **Self-Care Matters**: Prioritize your well-being and happiness. It's not selfish; it's essential for living your best life.

- **Positive Mindset**: Your perspective shapes your experience. Approach menopause with optimism and see it as an opportunity for growth.

- **Celebrate Your Achievements**: You've come a long way in life. Celebrate your accomplishments and look forward to new adventures.

Providing Additional Resources and Support

To further assist you in your menopausal journey, here are some additional resources and support avenues:

1. **Books**: Explore other books and literature dedicated to menopause and women's health for in-depth information and guidance. E.g *Intermittent Fasting and Exercise for Women By Daniel Watkins*, *Meals and Recipes for Women on Intermittent Fasting* and so many more.

2. **Online Communities**: Join online forums and communities where you can share experiences, ask questions, and gain support from other women.

3. **Professional Help:** Consult with healthcare providers, therapists, and counselors who specialize in women's health and menopause.

4. **Menopause Support Groups**: Seek out local or virtual menopause support groups in your area to connect with women who share your experiences.

5. **National and International Organizations**: Organizations such as the *North American Menopause Society* (NAMS) offer educational resources and support for women going through menopause.

With the knowledge and strategies provided in this guide and the support you can find through various resources, you have the tools to navigate menopause with grace and confidence. It's your time to shine, to embrace this incredible phase of life, and to celebrate the powerful, beautiful woman that you are.